CONTENTS

INTRODUCTION

With more than twelve years of experience in postgraduate medical education to draw on, PASTEST have commissioned a series of reasonably priced MCQ books under the editorial mantle of Dr Richard Hawkins.

There is no better way to revise for the MRCP Part I examination than by answering good quality MCQs. These books, however, provide an additional dimension. The MCQs have been deliberately broken down by specialty and a self-assessment chart provided for each so that doctors can identify their strengths and weaknesses and plan their revision accordingly.

A significant number of questions in the MRCP Part I examination are devoted to Rheumatology, Haematology and Infectious Diseases. This book provides approximately 34 representative questions from each specialty, with each question accompanied by a clear and simple explanatory answer. A strong emphasis on physiology, basic sciences and pharmacology has been included since the modern examination places such importance on these aspects.

The membership examination at present consists of sixty questions, each with a stem and five related questions: a total of 300 possible correct responses. Each correct response is awarded +1, each incorrect one -1, with no marks being awarded if the question is answered 'Don't know'. As in all examinations proper technique can make the difference between a 'pass' and a 'bare fail'.

What, then, is the best approach? Firstly, the question stem must be read very carefully. Failure to notice a negative statement could result in a score of -5. In a 'close marked' examination this could quite easily be the difference between a pass and a fail. Secondly, the keywords used in MCQs should be identified: always/commonly/frequently/recognised/may/never, and so on. Each has a distinctly different meaning, thus: 'jaundice is a frequent complication of infectious mononucleosis' (false), whereas: 'jaundice may complicate infectious mononucleosis' (true). Beware of always and never.

Finally, answer those questions that you think you have a greater than 50% chance of getting correct. Thus, while leaving out questions in which you would be guessing (because in these you are

PASTEST POCKET SERIES FOR MRCP PART 1

BOOK 4

MCQs IN RHEUMATOLOGY, HAEMATOLOGY AND INFECTIOUS DISEASES

Edited by Richard L. Hawkins MBBS FRCS

Authors: D. Macfarlane MD MRCP
D. O. Haskard MA MRCP
Lewisham and Guy's Hospitals,
London.

A. Yardumian MB MRCP
The Middlesex Hospital, London.

C. R. J. Singer BSc MB ChB MRCP
University College Hospital,
London.

J. Watson MB MSc MRCP
PHLS Communicable Disease
Surveillance Centre, London.

C. P. Conlan MB MRCP
University Teaching Hospital, Lusaka,
Zambia

PASTEST

Cranford Lodge, Bexton Road,
Knutsford, Cheshire. WA16 0ED
Telephone: 0565 55226

First printed 1987
Reprinted 1988
Reprinted 1989

British Library Cataloguing in Publication Data
Hawkins R.L.
MCQs in gastroenterology, endocrinology and
renal medicine.——(Pastest pocket book
series).
1. Medicine——Problems, exercises, etc.
610'.76 R834.5

ISBN: 0-906896-24-X

Text prepared by Turner Associates, Knutsford, Cheshire.
Phototypeset by Communitype, Leicester.
Printed by Martins, Berwick on Tweed.

likely to score 0 overall), do attempt those which you think you know something about; it is worth backing a hunch. Although your 'hit rate' will not be as high for these as for those questions for which you think you know the answer, overall you will score positively. Candidates do fail because they do not attempt enough questions, and it is worth remembering that even some of those answers that you are confident about may, in fact, be wrong.

Time for revision is often at a premium because preparation has to be done at the same time as a busy medical SHO job. A few general tips may be useful:

1. Do not read systematically through large medical textbooks, but rather base your revision around multiple choice questions. The self-assessment charts provided in this book may be helpful here. Direct further reading of standard texts to those areas in which you are scoring low marks, in other words use these MCQs to identify 'blind spots' in your knowledge.

2. Make cards for those questions which come up frequently (such as modes of inheritance) and learn these.

3. A good course is probably worth the investment and your employer may be able to assist with the funding for this, if one is not provided at your hospital.

4. Aim to start your revision in good time and be sure you have time to cover most topics.

Cut-out self-assessment charts are included in this book so that you can record your answers to each MCQ as you work steadily through the questions. In order to give yourself a realistic time limit, do not spend more than 2 ½ minutes on any one question. Some people may prefer to indicate their answers directly on the question pages in the spaces provided and then to transfer these answers on to the self-assessment charts. You can then correct your own answers against the answers given in the book and can calculate your total score in each section. By indicating clearly each item that you answered incorrectly you can then read the explanation provided and refer to a standard text book for further revision on that topic.

Encyclopaedic specialist reference books are perhaps best avoided during preparation, only to be used for verification of detail. However the following may prove useful to MRCP Candidates:

Dieppe, P. et al. **Rheumatological Medicine.** Churchill Livingstone.
Mandal, B.K. Mayon-White, R.T. **Lecture Notes on Infectious Diseases.** (4th edition) Blackwell Scientific.
Richards, Linch, Goldstone. **A Synopsis of Haematology.** Wright.

RHEUMATOLOGY SELF-ASSESSMENT CHART

Please use 2B PENCIL only. Rub out all errors thoroughly.
Mark lozenges like ⬬ NOT like this ⊄ ⊄ ⊄

T ⬭ = TRUE F ⬭ = FALSE DK ⬭ = DON'T KNOW

	A	B	C	D	E
1	T ⬭ F ⬭ DK ⬭	T ⬭ F ⬭ DK ⬭	T ⬭ F ⬭ DK ⬭	T ⬭ F ⬭ DK ⬭	T ⬭ F ⬭ DK ⬭
2	T ⬭ F ⬭ DK ⬭	T ⬭ F ⬭ DK ⬭	T ⬭ F ⬭ DK ⬭	T ⬭ F ⬭ DK ⬭	T ⬭ F ⬭ DK ⬭
3	T ⬭ F ⬭ DK ⬭	T ⬭ F ⬭ DK ⬭	T ⬭ F ⬭ DK ⬭	T ⬭ F ⬭ DK ⬭	T ⬭ F ⬭ DK ⬭
4	T ⬭ F ⬭ DK ⬭	T ⬭ F ⬭ DK ⬭	T ⬭ F ⬭ DK ⬭	T ⬭ F ⬭ DK ⬭	T ⬭ F ⬭ DK ⬭
5	T ⬭ F ⬭ DK ⬭	T ⬭ F ⬭ DK ⬭	T ⬭ F ⬭ DK ⬭	T ⬭ F ⬭ DK ⬭	T ⬭ F ⬭ DK ⬭
6	T ⬭ F ⬭ DK ⬭	T ⬭ F ⬭ DK ⬭	T ⬭ F ⬭ DK ⬭	T ⬭ F ⬭ DK ⬭	T ⬭ F ⬭ DK ⬭
7	T ⬭ F ⬭ DK ⬭	T ⬭ F ⬭ DK ⬭	T ⬭ F ⬭ DK ⬭	T ⬭ F ⬭ DK ⬭	T ⬭ F ⬭ DK ⬭
8	T ⬭ F ⬭ DK ⬭	T ⬭ F ⬭ DK ⬭	T ⬭ F ⬭ DK ⬭	T ⬭ F ⬭ DK ⬭	T ⬭ F ⬭ DK ⬭
9	T ⬭ F ⬭ DK ⬭	T ⬭ F ⬭ DK ⬭	T ⬭ F ⬭ DK ⬭	T ⬭ F ⬭ DK ⬭	T ⬭ F ⬭ DK ⬭
10	T ⬭ F ⬭ DK ⬭	T ⬭ F ⬭ DK ⬭	T ⬭ F ⬭ DK ⬭	T ⬭ F ⬭ DK ⬭	T ⬭ F ⬭ DK ⬭
11	T ⬭ F ⬭ DK ⬭	T ⬭ F ⬭ DK ⬭	T ⬭ F ⬭ DK ⬭	T ⬭ F ⬭ DK ⬭	T ⬭ F ⬭ DK ⬭
12	T ⬭ F ⬭ DK ⬭	T ⬭ F ⬭ DK ⬭	T ⬭ F ⬭ DK ⬭	T ⬭ F ⬭ DK ⬭	T ⬭ F ⬭ DK ⬭
13	T ⬭ F ⬭ DK ⬭	T ⬭ F ⬭ DK ⬭	T ⬭ F ⬭ DK ⬭	T ⬭ F ⬭ DK ⬭	T ⬭ F ⬭ DK ⬭
14	T ⬭ F ⬭ DK ⬭	T ⬭ F ⬭ DK ⬭	T ⬭ F ⬭ DK ⬭	T ⬭ F ⬭ DK ⬭	T ⬭ F ⬭ DK ⬭
15	T ⬭ F ⬭ DK ⬭	T ⬭ F ⬭ DK ⬭	T ⬭ F ⬭ DK ⬭	T ⬭ F ⬭ DK ⬭	T ⬭ F ⬭ DK ⬭

	A	B	C	D	E
16	T ⬭ F ⬭ DK ⬭	T ⬭ F ⬭ DK ⬭	T ⬭ F ⬭ DK ⬭	T ⬭ F ⬭ DK ⬭	T ⬭ F ⬭ DK ⬭
17	T ⬭ F ⬭ DK ⬭	T ⬭ F ⬭ DK ⬭	T ⬭ F ⬭ DK ⬭	T ⬭ F ⬭ DK ⬭	T ⬭ F ⬭ DK ⬭
18	T ⬭ F ⬭ DK ⬭	T ⬭ F ⬭ DK ⬭	T ⬭ F ⬭ DK ⬭	T ⬭ F ⬭ DK ⬭	T ⬭ F ⬭ DK ⬭
19	T ⬭ F ⬭ DK ⬭	T ⬭ F ⬭ DK ⬭	T ⬭ F ⬭ DK ⬭	T ⬭ F ⬭ DK ⬭	T ⬭ F ⬭ DK ⬭
20	T ⬭ F ⬭ DK ⬭	T ⬭ F ⬭ DK ⬭	T ⬭ F ⬭ DK ⬭	T ⬭ F ⬭ DK ⬭	T ⬭ F ⬭ DK ⬭
21	T ⬭ F ⬭ DK ⬭	T ⬭ F ⬭ DK ⬭	T ⬭ F ⬭ DK ⬭	T ⬭ F ⬭ DK ⬭	T ⬭ F ⬭ DK ⬭
22	T ⬭ F ⬭ DK ⬭	T ⬭ F ⬭ DK ⬭	T ⬭ F ⬭ DK ⬭	T ⬭ F ⬭ DK ⬭	T ⬭ F ⬭ DK ⬭
23	T ⬭ F ⬭ DK ⬭	T ⬭ F ⬭ DK ⬭	T ⬭ F ⬭ DK ⬭	T ⬭ F ⬭ DK ⬭	T ⬭ F ⬭ DK ⬭
24	T ⬭ F ⬭ DK ⬭	T ⬭ F ⬭ DK ⬭	T ⬭ F ⬭ DK ⬭	T ⬭ F ⬭ DK ⬭	T ⬭ F ⬭ DK ⬭
25	T ⬭ F ⬭ DK ⬭	T ⬭ F ⬭ DK ⬭	T ⬭ F ⬭ DK ⬭	T ⬭ F ⬭ DK ⬭	T ⬭ F ⬭ DK ⬭
26	T ⬭ F ⬭ DK ⬭	T ⬭ F ⬭ DK ⬭	T ⬭ F ⬭ DK ⬭	T ⬭ F ⬭ DK ⬭	T ⬭ F ⬭ DK ⬭
27	T ⬭ F ⬭ DK ⬭	T ⬭ F ⬭ DK ⬭	T ⬭ F ⬭ DK ⬭	T ⬭ F ⬭ DK ⬭	T ⬭ F ⬭ DK ⬭
28	T ⬭ F ⬭ DK ⬭	T ⬭ F ⬭ DK ⬭	T ⬭ F ⬭ DK ⬭	T ⬭ F ⬭ DK ⬭	T ⬭ F ⬭ DK ⬭
29	T ⬭ F ⬭ DK ⬭	T ⬭ F ⬭ DK ⬭	T ⬭ F ⬭ DK ⬭	T ⬭ F ⬭ DK ⬭	T ⬭ F ⬭ DK ⬭
30	T ⬭ F ⬭ DK ⬭	T ⬭ F ⬭ DK ⬭	T ⬭ F ⬭ DK ⬭	T ⬭ F ⬭ DK ⬭	T ⬭ F ⬭ DK ⬭

	A	B	C	D	E
31	T F DK	T F DK	T F DK	T F DK	T F DK
32	T F DK	T F DK	T F DK	T F DK	T F DK
33	T F DK	T F DK	T F DK	T F DK	T F DK

CORRECT ANSWERS (+1) =

INCORRECT ANSWERS (−1) =

DON'T KNOW (0) ______

TOTAL SCORE: ______

HAEMATOLOGY SELF-ASSESSMENT CHART

	A	B	C	D	E
34	T F DK	T F DK	T F DK	T F DK	T F DK
35	T F DK	T F DK	T F DK	T F DK	T F DK
36	T F DK	T F DK	T F DK	T F DK	T F DK
37	T F DK	T F DK	T F DK	T F DK	T F DK
38	T F DK	T F DK	T F DK	T F DK	T F DK
39	T F DK	T F DK	T F DK	T F DK	T F DK
40	T F DK	T F DK	T F DK	T F DK	T F DK
41	T F DK	T F DK	T F DK	T F DK	T F DK
42	T F DK	T F DK	T F DK	T F DK	T F DK
43	T F DK	T F DK	T F DK	T F DK	T F DK
44	T F DK	T F DK	T F DK	T F DK	T F DK
45	T F DK	T F DK	T F DK	T F DK	T F DK
46	T F DK	T F DK	T F DK	T F DK	T F DK
47	T F DK	T F DK	T F DK	T F DK	T F DK
48	T F DK	T F DK	T F DK	T F DK	T F DK
49	T F DK	T F DK	T F DK	T F DK	T F DK
50	T F DK	T F DK	T F DK	T F DK	T F DK
51	T F DK	T F DK	T F DK	T F DK	T F DK
52	T F DK	T F DK	T F DK	T F DK	T F DK
53	T F DK	T F DK	T F DK	T F DK	T F DK
54	T F DK	T F DK	T F DK	T F DK	T F DK
55	T F DK	T F DK	T F DK	T F DK	T F DK

	A	B	C	D	E
56	T F DK	T F DK	T F DK	T F DK	T F DK
57	T F DK	T F DK	T F DK	T F DK	T F DK
58	T F DK	T F DK	T F DK	T F DK	T F DK
59	T F DK	T F DK	T F DK	T F DK	T F DK
60	T F DK	T F DK	T F DK	T F DK	T F DK
61	T F DK	T F DK	T F DK	T F DK	T F DK
62	T F DK	T F DK	T F DK	T F DK	T F DK
63	T F DK	T F DK	T F DK	T F DK	T F DK
64	T F DK	T F DK	T F DK	T F DK	T F DK
65	T F DK	T F DK	T F DK	T F DK	T F DK
66	T F DK	T F DK	T F DK	T F DK	T F DK
67	T F DK	T F DK	T F DK	T F DK	T F DK
68	T F DK	T F DK	T F DK	T F DK	T F DK
69	T F DK	T F DK	T F DK	T F DK	T F DK

CORRECT ANSWERS (+1) =

INCORRECT ANSWERS (−1) =

DON'T KNOW (0) ____________

TOTAL SCORE: ____________

INFECTIOUS DISEASES SELF-ASSESSMENT CHART

	A	B	C	D	E
70	T F DK	T F DK	T F DK	T F DK	T F DK
71	T F DK	T F DK	T F DK	T F DK	T F DK
72	T F DK	T F DK	T F DK	T F DK	T F DK
73	T F DK	T F DK	T F DK	T F DK	T F DK
74	T F DK	T F DK	T F DK	T F DK	T F DK
75	T F DK	T F DK	T F DK	T F DK	T F DK
76	T F DK	T F DK	T F DK	T F DK	T F DK
77	T F DK	T F DK	T F DK	T F DK	T F DK
78	T F DK	T F DK	T F DK	T F DK	T F DK
79	T F DK	T F DK	T F DK	T F DK	T F DK

Infectious Diseases Continued

	A	B	C	D	E
80	T F DK	T F DK	T F DK	T F DK	T F DK
81	T F DK	T F DK	T F DK	T F DK	T F DK
82	T F DK	T F DK	T F DK	T F DK	T F DK
83	T F DK	T F DK	T F DK	T F DK	T F DK
84	T F DK	T F DK	T F DK	T F DK	T F DK
85	T F DK	T F DK	T F DK	T F DK	T F DK
86	T F DK	T F DK	T F DK	T F DK	T F DK
87	T F DK	T F DK	T F DK	T F DK	T F DK
88	T F DK	T F DK	T F DK	T F DK	T F DK
89	T F DK	T F DK	T F DK	T F DK	T F DK
90	T F DK	T F DK	T F DK	T F DK	T F DK
91	T F DK	T F DK	T F DK	T F DK	T F DK

	A	B	C	D	E
92	T F DK	T F DK	T F DK	T F DK	T F DK
93	T F DK	T F DK	T F DK	T F DK	T F DK
94	T F DK	T F DK	T F DK	T F DK	T F DK
95	T F DK	T F DK	T F DK	T F DK	T F DK
96	T F DK	T F DK	T F DK	T F DK	T F DK
97	T F DK	T F DK	T F DK	T F DK	T F DK
98	T F DK	T F DK	T F DK	T F DK	T F DK
99	T F DK	T F DK	T F DK	T F DK	T F DK
100	T F DK	T F DK	T F DK	T F DK	T F DK
101	T F DK	T F DK	T F DK	T F DK	T F DK
102	T F DK	T F DK	T F DK	T F DK	T F DK

CORRECT ANSWERS (+1) =

INCORRECT ANSWERS (−1) =

DON'T KNOW (0)

TOTAL SCORE:

RHEUMATOLOGY

Indicate your answers by putting T (True), F (False) or D (Don't know) in the spaces provided.

1. The diagnosis of septic arthritis rather than acute gout is suggested by the finding of

A a synovial fluid glucose concentration half that of a simultaneous blood sample
B a synovial fluid pH of 7.1
C a synovial fluid leucocyte count of 25 per microlitre
D a cloudy synovial fluid
E the presence of bacteria in the synovial fluid

Your answers: A.........B.........C.........D.........E.........

2. IgM rheumatoid factor

A reacts with the Fab component of IgG
B is synthesised by T cells
C fixes complement
D is the predominant rheumatoid factor assayed by the Rose-Waaler reaction
E is diagnostic of rheumatoid arthritis

Your answers: A.........B.........C.........D.........E.........

3. Activation of complement

A cannot occur without the participation of immunoglobulins
B results in increased capillary permeability
C protects cells from lysis by stabilising cell membranes
D does not occur in serum heated to 56°C for 30 minutes
E leads to the migration of neutrophils into sites of inflammation

Your answers: A.........B.........C.........D.........E.........

Answers overleaf

ANSWERS AND EXPLANATIONS

1. E

Septic arthritis can be difficult to distinguish from acute gout in the absence of positive microbiology. A-D are non-specific features of inflammation. Turbidity of synovial fluid is the result of the high leucocyte count. In fact the two conditions sometimes coexist and it is wise to perform microbiological analyses (e.g. Gram stain and culture) and a search for crystals on all highly inflammatory synovial fluids.

2. C D

Rheumatoid factors (RF) are immunoglobulins that react with the Fc component of IgG. Immunoglobulins are secreted by B (Bursa derived) lymphocytes and plasma cells. The ability to fix complement is a general feature of IgM, as is the ability to agglutinate erythrocytes coated with antigen. The Rose-Waaler reaction measures the ability of RF to agglutinate sheep erythrocytes that have been coated with rabbit IgG directed against sheep erythrocytes. IgG antibodies are much less effective at agglutinating antigen coated erythrocytes than IgM, and hence IgG RF is poorly measured by this test. RF are not specific for rheumatoid arthritis.

3. B D E

Complement activation by the 'alternative pathway' occurs in the absence of antibodies by hydrolysis of C3 to C3b by substances such as endotoxin. Increased capillary permeability is largely due to the release of histamine from mast cells in response to C3a and C5a. These factors are also chemotactic for neutrophils. Lysis of cells coated with complement is a function of the late complement components C8 and C9, which create holes in cell membranes. Heat treatment is the standard laboratory method for inactivating complement.

4. Childhood dermatomyositis

A is characteristically associated with malignancy
B may be complicated by calcification of muscles
C may cause death from renal failure
D can be excluded by a normal ESR
E may be present despite normal muscle enzymes

Your answers: A.........B.........C.........D.........E.........

5. The following statements are true:

A occipital headaches can occur in temporal arteritis
B corneal reflex loss may be an early sign of rheumatoid cervical myelopathy
C the nail-fold infarcts of rheumatoid vasculitis represent evidence of a life-threatening complication
D iron therapy is effective in correcting the anaemia of rheumatoid arthritis
E gold injections are usually given intra-articularly

Your answers: A.........B.........C.........D.........E.........

6. Carpal tunnel syndrome

A may present with pain in the forearm
B is associated with fasciculation of the small muscles of the hand
C is exacerbated by coughing and sneezing
D an underlying medical condition is usually present
E is common in diffuse eosinophilic fasciitis

Your answers: A.........B.........C.........D.........E.........

Answers overleaf

4. E

Malignancy is an association with adult but not childhood dermatomyositis. Renal failure is not a feature although the kidneys may be histologically abnormal. Skin, fascia, subcutaneous tissue and fat (but not muscle) may calcify. The ESR is not elevated in approximately half. If muscle enzymes are normal further investigations such as EMG and/or muscle biopsy are indicated.

5. A B

The occipital artery may be involved as well as the temporal in temporal arteritis. The loss of the corneal reflex is due to compression of the spinal tract of the Vth cranial nerve which reaches to the level of the atlanto-axial joint of the neck. Nail-fold vasculitis is benign and self-limiting. Iron therapy is ineffective, and may make inflammation worse. Gold is given intramuscularly.

6. A E

The pain of median nerve compression can radiate to the forearm and may even present as a painful shoulder. Fasciculation is not a feature especially not of the small muscles of the hand as they are innervated by the ulnar nerve. Exacerbation by raising CSF pressure on coughing suggests nerve root compression in the neck. An underlying condition is rarely present in practice: most cases occurring in middle-aged people are a combination of hardening of the flexor retinaculum plus a congenitally small tunnel.

7. Secondary (reactive) amyloidosis

A results from an inability to mount an acute phase response
B causes ulceration of the tongue
C characteristically presents as a glomerulonephritis
D only complicates rheumatic diseases in adults
E can be reversed by controlling the underlying disease

Your answers: A.........B.........C.........D.........E.........

8. In children

A ankylosing spondylitis characteristically presents with a stiff painful back
B psoriasis characteristically precedes the onset of psoriatic arthropathy
C peripheral arthritis characteristically presents after onset of inflammatory bowel disease
D with juvenile chronic arthritis iritis is associated with antinuclear antibodies
E Reiter's syndrome is unknown

Your answers: A.........B.........C.........D.........E.........

9. Interleukin-1 (IL-1)

A is a lymphocyte activating factor
B is an endogenous pyrogen
C inhibits fibroblast proliferation
D stimulates the synthesis of acute phase proteins in the liver
E is not synthesised by macrophages

Your answers: A.........B.........C.........D.........E.........

Answers overleaf

7. None are correct

Reactive amyloidosis occurs as a result of a prolonged acute phase response, particularly elevation of the serum amyloid A protein which in genetically predisposed individuals cannot be catabolised and so becomes deposited in tissues as fibrils. The tongue may be enlarged with amyloid but not ulcerated. It typically presents with nephrotic syndrome. It may occur in children as well as adults and is progressive and fatal despite good control of the underlying disease.

8. C D

Ankylosing spondylitis characteristically presents as a lower limb oligoarthritis in boys followed later by spinal involvement. In adults psoriasis usually occurs before the arthritis but the opposite trend occurs in children. Inflammatory bowel disease has usually been present for several years prior to the onset of arthritis. Iritis is associated with anti-nuclear antibodies. Although the sexually acquired forms of Reiter's syndrome are very unusual in children, the enteric forms are quite common.

9. A B D

IL-1 has many biological effects including A, B, and D. IL-1 also is chemotactic for lymphocytes, increases the thrombogenicity of the endothelial luminal surface, promotes leucocyte adhesion to endothelium by an action on endothelial cells, and stimulates fibroblast proliferation. IL-1 is synthesised by many cells, of which macrophages are amongst the most important. Other sources include Langerhans cells, dendritic cells, keratinocytes and endothelial cells.

10. The following statements about synovial fluid are true:

A it is often blood-stained in acute pyrophosphate arthropathy

B the greater the inflammation, the more viscous the fluid

C a turbid fluid indicates the presence of infection

D synovial fluid lactate levels are higher in infected than in non- infected effusions

E crystals may be visualised by holding a specimen against a dark background in natural daylight

Your answers: A.........B.........C.........D.........E.........

11. The delayed hypersensitivity reaction (Type IV)

A is a humoral immune response

B is dependent upon T lymphocytes

C is characterised by a mononuclear cell infiltration

D is caused by deposition of immune complexes in tissues

E is mediated by IgE antibodies bound to Fc receptors on mast cells and basophil granulocytes

Your answers: A.........B.........C.........D.........E.........

12. Sjögren's syndrome

A should be treated with topical steroid eye drops

B causes dyspareunia

C affects men more than women

D may cause facial swelling

E is associated with the Anti-SS-A antibody

Your answers: A.........B.........C.........D.........E.........

Answers overleaf

10. A D

Synovial inflammation is associated with release of proteolytic enzymes which degrade the hyaluronate making the fluid less viscous. A turbid fluid indicates the presence of white cells, not necessarily infection. Raised lactate levels are found in septic arthritis. Crystals of pyrophosphate and urate can be seen using polarised light microscopy. They are not visible to the naked eye.

11. B C

The delayed type hypersensitivity reaction (Type IV) is a T cell mediated response that results in a mononuclear cell infiltration into the site of antigen deposition. The cutaneous response to tuberculin purified protein derivative (PPD) is a typical example. Humoral antibodies are involved in types II and III hypersensitivity. In type II hypersensitivity, autoantibodies are directed against cell surface antigens, as in autoimmune haemolytic anaemia. In type III hypersensitivity, immune complexes are deposited in tissues, either in antibody excess (e.g. Farmer's lung) or in antigen excess (e.g. serum sickness). E refers to immediate (type I) hypersensitivity.

12. B D E

Steroid eye drops are not required and may be dangerous by predisposing to infection (particularly as a dry eye is prone to bacterial and fungal infection), scleral softening and perforation. The eye should be kept moist by regular use of artificial tears. Patients with some tear flow may benefit from electrocoagulation of the nasolacrimal glands to encourage the accumulation of residual tear drops. Other exocrine secretions, including those of the vagina, are affected, and the salivary glands may be enlarged typically in unilateral and episodic fashion. Most patients have the Anti- SS-A antibody named after the 'A' antigen of Sjögren's syndrome, now called anti-Ro.

? Duct

13. Raynaud's phenomenon

A may affect the tongue
B vasodilator drugs are beneficial
C is a feature of carpal tunnel syndrome
D is due to hyperviscosity of the blood
E should be treated with cytotoxic drugs

Your answers: A.........B.........C.........D.........E.........

14. In the drug treatment of rheumatoid arthritis the following may occur:

A heart failure with indomethacin
B proteinuria with azathioprine
C dermatomyositis with penicillamine
D myaesthenia gravis with gold
E rash with allopurinol

Your answers: A.........B.........C.........D.........E.........

15. Perthes' disease of the hip

A is the eponymous name given to a slipped femoral epiphysis
B is characteristically a disease of pubertal girls
C may present as a painless limp
D can be excluded on a plain radiograph
E fortunately does not affect both hips

Your answers: A.........B.........C.........D.........E.........

Answers overleaf

13. A

Raynaud's phenomenon may affect feet, tongue, and even the internal organs such as the kidney. It is not a feature of carpal tunnel syndrome and is due to hyper-reactivity of the digital blood vessels. Simple measures such as thermal gloves and avoidance of smoking and cold situations are all that is required for the majority. Vasodilator drugs such as nifedipine and prazosin have often been prescribed but are only occasionally beneficial.

14. A

Non-steroidal anti-inflammatory drugs may cause fluid retention and precipitate heart failure, particularly in the elderly. Renal side-effects do not occur with azathioprine. Penicillamine, not gold, may cause a myasthenia-like syndrome. Allopurinol has no place in the treatment of rheumatoid arthritis, although it may cause a rash.

15. C

Perthes' (also called Legg-Calvé-Perthes') disease is avascular necrosis of the femoral head and is a common disease of young boys (average age 7 years old). In 25% of cases it presents as a painless limp. Serial X-rays may be required to establish the diagnosis because the initial films are often normal. It is bilateral in about 10%.

16. In Henoch Schönlein purpura

A an erosive arthritis is recognised
B the purpuric lesions occur all together rather than in crops
C IgM is characteristically found in affected tissues on immunofluorescence
D low platelets cause gastrointestinal bleeding
E renal involvement is never severe

Your answers: A.........B.........C.........D.........E.........

17. The following are features of Lyme disease:

A erythema nodosum (EN)
B erythema chronicum migrans (ECM)
C arthritis clinically indistinguishable from juvenile chronic arthritis (JCA)
D Cranial nerve VII palsy
E responds to penicillin

Your answers: A.........B.........C.........D.........E.........

18. Juvenile chronic arthritis (JCA)

A is the same disease as adult rheumatoid arthritis (RA)
B there is a high incidence of uveitis in those with a negative antinuclear factor
C may result in blindness
D can present as PUO
E is characteristically associated with a bad long-term outlook

Your answers: A.........B.........C.........D.........E.........

Answers overleaf

16. None are correct

The arthritis is not erosive and complete recovery is the norm. The spots may occur in crops and relapses are common. IgA is characteristically found in the vessel walls. The platelets are normal although bleeding does occur due to vasculitis in the gut. Renal involvement occurs in about 50% of cases and can be very severe although this is uncommon (less than 10%). Glomerulonephritis is the characteristic lesion presenting either with symptomless proteinuria or haematoma or with nephrotic syndrome.

17. B C D E

The disease was first described (in 1975) because of close clustering of cases round the small community of Lyme, Connecticut. The disease is caused by a spirochaete-like organism called *Borrelia burgdorfi* and occurs world-wide. ECM characteristically starts at the site of the tick bite and spreads outwards as a bright red expanding circle with a pale centre. Originally affected children were thought to have juvenile chronic arthritis although neurological and cardiac features are more common. Neurological abnormalities include cranial nerve palsies, sensory radiculopathy and lymphocytic meningitis.

18. C D

Only 5% of children with JCA have RA, the remainder have distinct separate illnesses. JCA is divided by mode of onset into systemic, poly- and pauciarticular forms. Chronic uveitis occurs particularly in those with positive antinuclear factor and may cause insidious loss of vision. The systemic form (also called Still's disease) characteristically presents with a high swinging pyrexia. The majority of children recover and function well as adults.

19. Heberden's nodes

A are often associated with pain in the first metatarso-phalangeal joint
B may be associated with mucoid cysts
C are not inherited
D may regress following paralysis of a limb
E may be associated with synovitis, erosion and ankylosis

Your answers: A.........B.........C.........D.........E.........

20. Monosodium urate (MSU) crystals

A are weakly positively birefringent
B are rhomboidal
C are found within neutrophils in the synovial fluid in acute gout
D are water soluble
E can stimulate interleukin-1 (IL-1) secretion

Your answers: A.........B.........C.........D.........E.........

21. Osteomalacia

A is associated with a myopathy
B causes reduced bone volume
C must be corrected by using the more potent forms of vitamin D such as 1-alpha hydroxycholecalciferol
D may result in tertiary hyperparathyroidism
E causes lesions that are undetectable on bone scintigraphy

Your answers: A.........B.........C.........D.........E.........

Answers overleaf

19. A B D E

Primary generalised nodal osteoarthritis is inherited as a dominant trait in women and a recessive in men. The pattern of involvement is proximal and distal interphalangeal joints of the fingers, carpometacarpal joint of the thumb, cervical and lumbar spine, and metatarsophalangeal joint of the great toe. Small gelatinous cysts may occur near Heberden's nodes which contain pure hyaluronic acid. Limb paralysis following a stroke, for example, may result in significant regression of pre-existing nodes. There is a subset of osteoarthritis in which there is erosive destruction of the interphalangeal joints in association with Heberden's nodes, without the other features of generalised nodal osteoarthritis.

20. C D E

MSU crystals are strongly negatively birefringent and needle shaped. A and B refer to calcium pyrophosphate crystals which are responsible for chondrocalcinosis and pseudogout. The presence of intracellular MSU crystals in inflammatory fluid is diagnostic of acute gout. MSU is very water soluble, which should be considered when diluting or preserving pathological material. The secretion of IL-1 from monocytes in response to MSU crystals may play an important role in the pathophysiology of acute gout.

21. A D

Muscle weakness and tenderness are quite common and may contribute to the characteristic waddling gait. The bone volume is normal but undercalcified. The more potent forms of vitamin D are not required since uncomplicated osteomalacia is due to dietary deficiency and is therefore not resistant to treatment. The potent forms can be dangerous resulting in hypercalcaemia. Prolonged hypocalcaemia results in secondary hyperparathyroidism which can occasionally become autonomous. The bone scan is a useful way of detecting lesions since the decalcified bones avidly take up bone-seeking isotopes.

22. Leucocytes of the CD4 (T4) phenotype

A are lymphocytes
B do not recirculate
C are phagocytic
D are infected by the Human Immunodeficiency Virus (HIV)
E perform a 'helper' role in the on-going immune response

Your answers: A.........B.........C.........D.........E.........

23. The following are true of Paget's disease:

A internal hydrocephalus may occur
B joint replacement surgery is contraindicated because of poor bone healing
C parathormone concentration is elevated
D although the serum calcium is normal, the urinary calcium is elevated
E it is rare for both articulating surfaces of an affected joint to be affected

Your answers: A.........B.........C.........D.........E.........

24. Anti-histone antibodies

A are associated with thrombosis
B are found in the absence of antibodies to native DNA in drug induced SLE
C are associated with congenital heart block
D are a marker for polymyositis
E are not found in rheumatoid arthritis

Your answers: A.........B.........C.........D.........E.........

Answers overleaf

22. A D E

The T4 antigen, now designated CD4 (CD=cluster of differentiation), is a marker for a subpopulation of T lymphocytes that are thought to play a 'helper' role in the immune response. Long-lived resting lymphocytes enter lymphoid tissue, such as lymph nodes, and pass through the lymphoid parenchyma into efferent lymph. Thence the lymphocytes pass into the central lymphatic ducts and then back into the blood stream. This process of lymphocyte migration is called recirculation and allows each individual lymphoid organ to share the large pool of recirculating lymphocytes with the rest of the immune system, thus disseminating immunological function and memory. Most small resting T lymphocytes are considered to be recirculating cells. HIV preferentially infects T4 cells and may enter the cell by way of the T4 antigen.

23. A

Basilar invagination occurs when the soft skull base descends over the top of the spinal cord. This can obstruct the flow of cerebrospinal fluid and cause hydrocephalus. Bone healing, whether after a fracture or following surgery, is either completely normal or at worst slightly delayed and Paget's disease is therefore not a contraindication to surgery. The parathormone level is normal, and if found elevated, suggests the presence of coexistent hyperparathyroidism. Both surfaces of a joint may be involved, particularly in the hip joint, resulting in pagetic coxarthropathy. The joint space may be preserved early on but with progressive deformity of the softened femoral head, secondary degenerative changes supervene.

24. B

Although anti-histone antibodies are found in 30-80% of sera from patients with idiopathic SLE, their presence in patients with clinical SLE who lack antibodies to native DNA is suggestive of a drug induced syndrome. Anti-histone antibodies are found in 15-20% of patients with rheumatoid arthritis and are therefore only diagnostically valuable in the appropriate clinical setting. A refers to anti-cardiolipin antibodies. C refers to antibodies to the Ro (SS-A) antigen. D refers to antibodies to the Jo-1 antigen.

25. In acute gout

A the serum urate is always elevated
B the attack only settles once all the crystals have been removed from the synovial fluid by phagocytosis
C the presence of fever, raised ESR and raised white cell count means the diagnosis is incorrect
D colchicine no longer has a therapeutic role
E only one joint is affected at any one time

Your answers: A.........B.........C.........D.........E.........

26. The following statements are true:

A radiological sacroiliitis is characteristically unilateral in ankylosing spondylitis
B periostitis is a frequent radiological finding in psoriatic arthropathy
C juxta-articular osteoporosis does not occur with gouty erosions
D erosions are characteristically periarticular in systemic lupus erythematosus (SLE)
E gouty tophi are radio-opaque

Your answers: A.........B.........C.........D.........E.........

27. The following are recognised features of Wegener's granulomatosis:

A loss of hearing
B corneal ulceration
C impaired oesophageal motility
D collapse of the bridge of the nose
E asymptomatic pulmonary lesions

Your answers: A.........B.........C.........D.........E.........

Answers overleaf

25. None are correct

Although sustained hyperuricaemia is a necessary prerequisite for developing gout, during the acute attack the level may fall to normal. The finding of negatively birefringent crystals in synovial fluid on polarised light microscopy confirms the diagnosis but repeat examination of the fluid after the acute attack has subsided may still reveal crystals which are rendered non-inflammatory. Acute crystal synovitis induces an acute phase response of which fever, leucocytosis and raised ESR are a part. The only sure way to exclude joint sepsis is to culture the fluid. 90% of all attacks are monoarticular but 10% affect more than one joint. High doses of NSAIDs e.g. indomethacin 100 mg stat, followed by 50 mg every 6 hours are extremely effective in treating the acute attack. However, colchicine is still a useful alternative, particularly for those on anticoagulants or with a history of peptic ulceration.

26. B C

Sacroiliitis is characteristically bilateral and symmetrical in ankylosing spondylitis. Unilateral, asymmetrical involvement is more common in other forms of seronegative spondarthritis such as psoriasis and Reiter's syndrome. Fluffy periostitis often occurs in conjunction with erosions in psoriatic arthropathy, so-called proliferative erosions. SLE is a non-erosive arthropathy and although there may be considerable hand deformity, this is due to tendon involvement rather than joint destruction. Gouty tophi do not calcify as a rule and are therefore radiolucent. The bone density around gouty erosions is usually normal although during an acute attack of gout there may be osteoporosis in the affected joint.

27. A B D E

Serous otitis media is common and occurs early in Wegener's granulomatosis and often results in loss of hearing. The granulomatous vasculitis, which is the characteristic pathological lesion, can affect the tissues of the eye resulting in scleritis, episcleritis and corneal ulceration. The granulomatous tissue is able to erode cartilage and this can produce collapse of the bridge of the nose. The disease characteristically starts in the upper airways, but the lower respiratory tract is usually involved eventually, presenting as cough or haemoptysis, or may be detected as asymptomatic pulmonary infiltrates on a chest X-ray. Impaired oesophageal motility is a feature of the scleroderma group of illnesses.

28. The following are characteristically involved:

A the MCP joints in psoriatic arthropathy
B the hip in ankylosing spondylitis
C the DIP joints in pyrophosphate arthropathy
D the MTP joints in haemophilia
E the hand and foot in sickle cell disease

Your answers: A.........B.........C.........D.........E.........

29. On neurological examination of the musculoskeletal system the following pairs are correct:

A weak wrist flexion: C6/C7
B weak thumb extension: C7/C8
C weak thumb adduction: C8/TI
D absent knee jerk: L5
E weak dorsiflexion of the big toe: L5/SI

Your answers: A.........B.........C.........D.........E.........

30. The following are recognised features of rheumatoid arthritis (RA):

A exacerbation during pregnancy
B iritis
C dry mouth
D sacroiliitis
E leg ulceration

Your answers: A.........B.........C.........D.........E.........

Answers overleaf

28. B E

There are several characteristic patterns of joint involvement in psoriasis: 1. DIP joint disease in association with nail dystrophy (10%); 2. asymmetrical oligoarticular involvement of the small distal joints (70%); 3. symmetrical polyarthritis (15%); 4. axial with spondylitis as a major feature (5%); 5. arthritis mutilans (rare). Generally, a seronegative oligoarthritis with DIP and PIP involvement with relative sparing of the MCP joints suggests a diagnosis of psoriatic arthritis. Extraspinal joint involvement occurs in 40% of patients with ankylosing spondylitis, the hip and knee being the commonest sites. Pyrophosphate deposition occurs mainly in the large joints, particularly the knees, wrists and shoulders. The joints involved in haemophilia (in order of frequency) are the knee, elbow, ankle, shoulder, wrist and sternoclavicular joint. Acute pain and swelling of a digit or a whole extremity is characteristic of multiple bone infarction in children during a sickle crisis.

29. A B C

30. C E

RA is usually improved during pregnancy due to the increase of pregnancy-associated globulin which has anti-inflammatory properties. Iritis occurs no more frequently than in the general population and is not one of the common types of eye lesions found in RA. Dry mouth is a component of Sjögren's or sicca syndrome which occurs in many patients with RA. Pathologically there is lymphocytic infiltration of the lacrimal and salivary secretory tissue. Sacroiliitis is not a feature of RA. Leg ulcers which are slow-healing are common. Some, but not all, are due to vasculitis. Poor tissue healing and the effects of drugs are also thought to be factors.

31. The rash of systemic juvenile chronic arthritis (JCA):

A is raised, red and scaly
B characteristically comes and goes
C may be brought out by a hot bath
D is a photosensitivity rash
E is an extremely useful diagnostic sign

Your answers: A.........B.........C.........D.........E.........

32. The following are characteristic of polymyalgia rheumatica (PMR):

A depression
B weight loss
C lymphadenopathy
D raised muscle enzymes
E sternoclavicular joint swelling

Your answers: A.........B.........C.........D.........E.........

33. In systemic lupus erythematosus (SLE)

A the diagnosis should not be considered in the absence of antinuclear antibodies (ANA)
B a false positive VDRL test may indicate increased risk of neuropsychiatric involvement
C idiopathic thrombocytopenia purpura (ITP) is a recognised presentation in children
D pregnancy is contraindicated
E antibodies to double-stranded DNA cross the placenta and may cause congenital heart block

Your answers: A.........B.........C.........D.........E.........

Answers overleaf

31. B C E

Faced with a child with a PUO, the rash of systemic JCA is so characteristic that its recognition by an experienced observer can help make the diagnosis. It is salmon-pink, macular, and may literally appear and disappear within minutes. It often appears at a time when the temperature starts to rise and a hot bath may bring it out but sunlight has no effect. In a child with joint disease, a raised scaly rash should suggest psoriasis, and a photosensitive rash systemic lupus erythematosus.

32. A B E

The typical features of PMR outside the musculoskeletal system are depression and weight loss. There may also be low-grade fever. If temporal arteritis supervenes there may also be headache and facial pain. The presence of lymphadenopathy should alert one to the possibility of a paraneoplastic syndrome, which may present with similar clinical features. Muscle enzymes are raised in polymyositis which is associated with muscle fibril destruction. It is increasingly recognised that there may be synovitis in patients with PMR particularly affecting the shoulders and sterno-clavicular joints. Occasionally there may also be peripheral synovitis in the small joints of the hands resembling rheumatoid arthritis.

33. B C

ANA-negative SLE is increasingly recognised and presents mainly with skin disease. The tests for antibodies to double-stranded DNA and soluble nuclear antigens, particularly Ro (or SAA) are often positive. Antiphospholipid antibodies are found in some patients with SLE and may give a false positive VDRL test for syphilis. Such antibodies are associated with an increased risk of thrombosis, fetal wastage and neuro-psychiatric disease. Some children with ITP develop SLE as they grow up. Pregnancy is no longer contraindicated in lupus except in those with severe renal disease, although achieving conception may be more difficult and there is an increased incidence of miscarriage. Anti-Ro antibodies can cross the placenta and cause congenital heart block.

HAEMATOLOGY

Indicate your answers by putting T (True), F (False) or D (Don't know) in the spaces provided.

34. Vitamin B_{12}

A is found in meat, dairy products and green leaf vegetables
B stores in the body are adequate for about 3 years if intake ceases
C deficiency due to pernicious anaemia is rare in Africa and Asia
D deficiency can impair absorption of vitamin B_{12} itself
E requires replacement in patients on regular haemodialysis for renal disease

Your answers: A.........B.........C.........D.........E.........

35. Hairy cell leukaemia (HCL)

A is usually associated with splenomegaly
B is usually associated with an atypical lymphocytosis in the peripheral blood
C is usually a T-cell neoplasm
D is often controlled by splenectomy
E responds to interferon in the majority of patients

Your answers: A.........B.........C.........D.........E.........

36. The O_2 dissociation curve for adult haemoglobin

A is shifted to the right by 2,3-diphosphoglycerate (2,3DPG)
B is to the left of the O_2 dissociation curve of haemoglobin for the normal neonate at birth
C is shifted to the left in pyruvate kinase deficiency
D is shifted to the right in glucose-6-phosphate dehydrogenase (G6PD) deficiency
E is shifted to the left in Hb Chesapeake

Your answers: A.........B.........C.........D.........E.........

Answers overleaf

34. B C D

Vitamin B_{12} is synthesised soley by micro-organisms; the only source in the human diet is food of animal origin, (especially liver and kidney). All vegetable food is free of B_{12}. The body stores of the vitamin (2-3 mg) are sufficient for 3-4 years, as daily requirements are very low normally, in the order of 1-3 μg. Pernicious anaemia is the commonest megaloblastic anaemia in north Europeans, but rare in Asians and Africans. Deficiency of the vitamin does cause an ileal absorptive defect, and can impair its own absorption even if the deficiency is due to dietary causes. For this reason, Schilling tests should be delayed for about 6 weeks after starting parenteral treatment. B_{12} is firmly protein bound, unlike folate, and so is not removed during dialysis.

35. A D E

HCL usually presents with moderate splenomegaly and removal of the spleen often controls the disease for a period of months to years. While there are frequently atypical 'hairy cells' in the peripheral blood, lymphocytosis is uncommon. The marrow at presentation may contain numerous hairy cells, but the blood picture is usually one of pancytopenia. By far the majority of cases are B-cell neoplasms, but occasional cases with a T- lymphocyte phenotype have been described. Interferon does seem to induce remission in most patients but relapse commonly occurs after treatment is stopped.

36. A B E

By bonding to the haemoglobin molecule and fixing it in a low O_2 affinity configuration, 2,3 DPG shifts the O_2 dissociation curve to the right and increases O_2 delivery to the tissues. This occurs as a compensatory mechanism in many chronic anaemias. In utero and at birth the O_2 affinity of fetal blood is increased compared to that of adult haemoglobin, but shortly after birth the 2,3 DPG rises and becomes the same as that of adult blood. Deficiency of pyruvate kinase in the glycolytic pathway leads to accumulation of 2,3 DPG in the red cells and therefore shifts the curve to the right, but G6PD deficiency has no effect on 2,3 DPG levels or the O_2 dissociation curve. Chesapeake is the most common haemoglobinopathy to have increased oxygen affinity.

37. Immune thrombocytopenic purpura (ITP)

A can be diagnosed from a low platelet count plus appropriate bone marrow findings
B is usually associated with a palpable spleen
C should be treated with steroids in the first instance in patients over the age of 2
D usually runs a protracted indolent course in childhood
E may be induced by quinine sulphate

Your answers: A.........B.........C.........D.........E.........

38. Lymphocytosis

A in chronic lymphocytic leukaemia (CLL) may be due to T-cell proliferation
B in pertussis morphologically resembles CLL
C presenting in association with skin rashes is frequently of T-cell origin
D in glandular fever resembles that of CLL
E is a racial variant occurring not uncommonly in people of African origin

Your answers: A.........B.........C.........D.........E.........

39. Dietary iron

A in a normal diet amounts to about 3 mg per day
B absorption is reduced by vitamin C
C absorption is reduced by phosphates
D is about 90% excreted in health
E is absorbed in the ferric (Fe^{3+}) state

Your answers: A.........B.........C.........D.........E.........

Answers overleaf

37. E

The combination of thrombocytopenia and increased numbers of megakaryocytes in the marrow is characteristic of ITP, but can also occur in other, non-immune consumptive causes of thrombocytopenia e.g. splenomegaly, DIC. A palpable spleen is uncommon in ITP. While steroids are usually the first-line treatment in adults, in children treatment is frequently unnecessary but if it becomes imperative (clinical bleeding or platelet count less than 20 x 10^9/l) intravenous immunoglobulin is the treatment of choice. In children the disease is usually brief and self-limiting; it may follow a viral illness. Many drugs, including quinine, quinidine, para-aminosalicylic acid, rifampicin and sulphonamides may give rise to the syndrome.

38. A B C

Classical CLL is a lymphocyte proliferation usually of B cells which chiefly look small and 'mature' morphologically. Less commonly surface markers reveal a T-cell phenotype. The peripheral blood film in whooping cough may closely resemble CLL. Some chronic skin conditions (e.g. photosensitive eczema) may show circulating Sezary-like cells, and the T-cell lymphoproliferative disorders (mycosis fungoides/Sezary syndrome) frequently present to the dermatologist. In infectious mononucleosis the lymphocytes are of very different morphology, being large with plentiful cytoplasm, they resemble monocytes or sometimes blast cells. Neutropenia is a fairly frequent finding in Africans so that a 'reversed differential' (lymphocytes-neutrophils) may be found but an absolute lymphocytosis cannot be accounted for by this alone.

39. C D

The normal diet contains 10-15 mg of elemental iron per day; for absorption it must be reduced to the ferrous (Fe^{2+}) state. Vitamin C is a reducing substance and therefore enhances conversion to Fe^{2+} and absorption of the element, but phosphates can form insoluble complexes with iron and impair absorption. In health, only about 10% of iron ingested is absorbed, this can increase to 30% in iron depletion.

40. The following statements are true about Factor VIII:

A it consists of two parts of approximately equal size

B synthesis of Factor VIIIc and VIII von Willebrand factor (VWF) is controlled by sex-linked (X chromosomes) genes

C synthesis of VIIIc and VWF takes place chiefly in the liver

D in von Willebrand's disease, there is a reduction in both VIIIc and VIII VWF

E a factor VIIIc level of 10% (normal range 50-150%) is associated with a severe bleeding diathesis

Your answers: A.........B.........C.........D.........E.........

41. The incidence of acute leukaemia is increased in

A Down's syndrome

B Kleinfelter's syndrome

C ataxia telangiectasia

D Fanconi's anaemia

E Hodgkin's disease

Your answers: A.........B.........C.........D.........E.........

42. In a patient with paroxysmal nocturnal haemoglobinuria (PNH)

A iron may precipitate acute haemolysis

B aplastic anaemia is a recognised complication

C chronic granulocytic leukaemia may supervene

D the Hess test is commonly abnormal

E splenomegaly is commonly present

Your answers: A.........B.........C.........D.........E.........

Answers overleaf

40. D

Factor VIIIc, the factor taking part in the intrinsic clotting cascade is very much smaller than the large, polymerised factor VIII VWF, which acts as a carrier molecule. VIII VWF is under autosomal genetic control (so that both sexes can suffer from von Willebrand's disease); VIIIc is sex-linked. VIII VWF is synthesised chiefly by endothelial cells, the site of VIIIc synthesis is not clear; all the other clotting factors are synthesised in the liver. The primary problem in von Willebrand's disease is reduction in the level of VIII VWF, but VIIIc is also reduced, either because its stability is reduced when it is not complexed to VIII VWF or because VIII VWF in some way controls the rate of synthesis of VIIIc. Severe haemophilia A only really occurs at an VIIIc level of 1% or less; 10% would usually be associated with a relatively mild bleeding diathesis.

41. A B C D E

The risk of acute leukaemia is increased in all these conditions. Down's syndrome is characteristically associated with acute lymphoblastic leukaemia though acute myeloblastic anaemia (AML) is also more common in older patients. Fanconi's anaemia is in contrast characteristically associated with AML. Secondary leukaemia (usually AML) is a complication of alkylating agents and radiotherapy used in the treatment of Hodgkin's disease.

42. A B

Iron may indeed precipitate haemolysis and this is a not uncommon presenting feature. The mechanism may be due to increased output of complement sensitive reticulocytes following iron treatment in patients with marginal iron balance. Aplastic anaemia may supervene but there is no association with chronic granulocytic leukaemia. The Ham's acidified serum test is positive in PNH but the Hess test is not commonly abnormal unless thrombocytopenia occurs due to progressive aplasia. Splenomegaly is unusual.

43. Human lymphocyte

A T cells are considerably more numerous than B cells in peripheral blood
B T cells form ‘rosettes’ with mouse erythrocytes
C B cells mature in the bone marrow in mammals
D B cells are found in lymph node follicles
E T cells are found in the germinal centre of lymph node follicles

Your answers: A.........B.........C.........D.........E.........

44. The following are consistent with a diagnosis of ‘benign monoclonal gammopathy’ (BMG):

A Bence-Jones protein
B osteolytic lesions on X-ray
C 5% plasma cells in the bone marrow
D elevated serum calcium
E biclonal gammopathy

Your answers: A.........B.........C.........D.........E.........

45. A prolonged thrombin clotting time may occur in

A warfarin therapy
B prothrombin deficiency
C disseminated intravascular coagulation (DIC)
D dysfibrinogenaemia
E liver disease

Your answers: A.........B.........C.........D.........E.........

Answers overleaf

43. A C D

Approximately 70% of the total peripheral blood lymphocytes in humans are T cells, 10-20% are B cells and there are some 'null' cells. T lymphocytes form rosettes with sheep erythrocytes, this is how they are typed; it is the cells of classical chronic lymphocytic leukaemia which rosette mouse erythrocytes. The marrow appears to be the site of B cell maturation in mammals; the thymus is that of T cell maturation. B cells comprise the main population of lymph node follicles, situated in the node cortex. After antigenic challenge secondary follicles form, with a mantle of small B cells and a germinal centre which does not contain T cells but seems to be important in B cell memory. T cells are chiefly confined to the paracortical area, more deeply situated in the node.

44. A C E

Bence-Jones protein may occasionally occur in BMG and does not per se indicate multiple myeloma. Biclonal gammopathy, though uncommon, may occasionally occur in either BMG or multiple myeloma. 5% plasma cells may occur as a reactive feature and are not uncommon in the bone marrow of older patients. In contrast, osteolytic lesions and an elevated serum calcium are highly suggestive of multiple myeloma.

45. C D E

The thrombin time tests only the conversion of fibrinogen to fibrin by the addition of thrombin to citrated plasma. It is only prolonged as a result of absent, deficient or dysfunctional fibrinogen (as in liver disease) or in the presence of inhibitors, i.e. heparin or fibrinogen degradation products (as in DIC).

46. In blood coagulation

A the intrinsic pathway proceeds more rapidly than the extrinsic one
B the intrinsic system is activated by blood coming into contact with a non-endothelialised surface e.g. subendothelium
C calcium ions are required for the intrinsic, but not the extrinsic pathway to proceed
D platelets play a part in the normal coagulation cascade
E when the coagulation mechanisms are working normally, blood may take more than an hour to clot in a dry, plastic tube

Your answers: A.........B.........C.........D.........E.........

47. Increased plasma erythropoietin occurs in

A aplastic anaemia
B polycythaemia rubra vera (PRV)
C renal failure
D massive obesity
E hepatoma

Your answers: A.........B.........C.........D.........E.........

48. The following features favour the diagnosis of adult leukaemia- lymphoma syndrome:

A West Indian origin
B positive HTLVIII serology
C Japanese origin
D hypocalcaemia
E rapidly progressive disease

Your answers: A.........B.........C.........D.........E.........

Answers overleaf

46. B D E

The 'intrinsic pathway' is more important physiologically than the extrinsic pathway and is activated by contact with non-endothelialised surfaces e.g. damaged vessel wall or prosthetic valves. It is slower than the 'extrinsic pathway' which is activated by a variety of tissue thromboplastins. Both pathways plus the 'common pathway' they lead to require calcium ions to proceed normally. The reactions involved in the intrinsic and common pathways usually take place on, and are catalysed by, platelet membrane phospholipids. Whole blood clotting time of a venous sample in a dry tube is not recommended as even the roughest guide to 'clotting ability' as it depends so much on the precise conditions e.g. temperature, trauma of venepuncture but especially on the material of the container. In plastic it may take an hour or more to clot; in glass this occurs much more quickly.

47. A D E

Increased plasma erythropoietin levels occur 'appropriately' in aplastic anaemia in an attempt to compensate for the failure of red cell production, and in massive obesity due to the hypoxia associated with hypoventilation. Inappropriate production is thought to be the mechanism in hepatoma. In PRV and renal failure, low levels are usually found.

48. A C E

Adult leukaemia-lymphoma syndrome is one of the few human neoplasms with an established viral aetiology, and is most commonly seen in either West Indian or Japanese patients. The virus HTLVI is the aetiological agent causing neoplastic proliferation of CD4 positive T-lymphocytes. Hypercalcaemia is common and rapid clinical deterioration is usual.

49. Regarding human blood groups

A naturally occurring anti-A and anti-B antibodies can be IgM and IgG
B most people secrete their A or B blood group antigens in saliva
C the ABO type of an individual can 'change' during some illnesses e.g. acute leukaemia
D group O is the commonest blood group in all racial groups
E lack of certain blood group antigens protects against *Plasmodium vivax*

Your answers: A.........B.........C.........D.........E.........

50. Thrombocytopenia is a recognised side-effect of the following drugs:

A aspirin
B oxymethalone
C thiazide diuretics
D gold
E dapsone

Your answers: A.........B.........C.........D.........E.........

51. In aplastic anaemia

A a history of preceding hepatitis A is associated with a relatively benign course
B immunosuppressive therapy may be effective
C a leuko-erythroblastic blood picture may be present at diagnosis
D ferrokinetic studies show predominant accumulation of isotope in the liver
E a positive Ham's test may be present

Your answers: A.........B.........C.........D.........E.........

Answers overleaf

49. A B C E

Naturally occurring anti-A and anti-B antibodies, which develop after the neonatal period, are chiefly IgM but IgG is usually detectable too. By contrast 'immune' antibodies raised after antigenic change are chiefly IgG. 80% of the population are secretors and excrete blood group antigens into saliva, sweat and tears. The A and B antigens can 'weaken' significantly during acute leukaemia sometimes to such an extent that they are no longer detectable. Group O (Rhesus 'D' positive) is the commonest group in Europeans, but there are wide racial variations, and in some groups A is commonest. Red cells that do not possess the minor blood group antigens Duffy a and b are resistant to invasion by P. vivax. Duffy a neg, b neg is an uncommon phenotype in Europeans, but occurs in about three quarters of Negro people.

50. C D

Aspirin's antiplatelet effect is mediated through cyclo-oxygenase inhibition, by irreversible acetylation; it does not cause thrombocytopenia. Oxymethalone may occasionally cause a rise in the platelet count in patients with aplastic anaemia. Thiazide and gold both cause thrombocytopenia, the former by increased consumption and the latter by this mechanism or marrow suppression. Dapsone may cause haemolysis but thrombocytopenia is not a recognised side-effect.

51. B D E

Hepatitis A may result in a serious, frequently profound aplasia with a serious outlook. At least some cases of aplastic anaemia are due to an immunological mechanism and may respond to anti-lymphocyte globulin. A leuko-erythroblastic film is not associated with aplastic anaemia but with marrow fibrosis or infiltration. An injection of Fe^{59} results in slow clearance of isotope from the plasma and most of the radioactivity accumulates in the liver, only a very small amount appearing in the erythrocytes. Paroxysmal nocturnal haemoglobinuria is associated with aplasia and Ham's test may be positive.

52. In glucose-6-phosphate dehydrogenase (G6PD) deficiency

A inheritance is autosomal recessive
B the syndrome is characteristically less severe in African than in Mediterranean populations
C the red cells in heterozygotes all show about half the normal enzyme activity
D haemolysis may be induced by aspirin
E Heinz bodies may be seen during a haemolytic crisis

Your answers: A.........B.........C.........D.........E.........

53. Cryoprecipitate

A is prepared by thawing fresh frozen plasma
B is free of the risk of hepatitis infection
C is rich in fibrinogen
D may reverse the platelet defect in uraemic patients
E is of therapeutic value in haemophilia B

Your answers: A.........B.........C.........D.........E.........

54. In multiple myeloma

A a characteristic feature is elevated serum calcium and alkaline phosphatase, but normal serum phosphate
B bone scans are usually unhelpful in establishing the extent of skeletal involvement
C intravenous pyelograms (IVP) are contraindicated due to the risk of renal impairment
D infection is the commonest cause of death
E the urinary β_2 microglobulin is a helpful parameter in the assessment of response to therapy

Your answers: A.........B.........C.........D.........E.........

Answers overleaf

52. B E

Inheritance of G6PD deficiency is X-linked recessive and heterozygous females have red cells with either fully normal enzyme activity or completely deficient activity due to inactivation of the X chromosome (the Lyon hypothesis). The deficiency commonly found in Africans is usually less severe than in Mediterraneans and 'favism' is rare in this population. Aspirin does not induce an oxidant stress on the red cells and is not implicated in the haemolysis, which is associated with the presence of Heinz bodies due to denatured haemoglobin.

53. A C D

Cryoprecipitate is formed by thawing fresh frozen plasma from a recent donation and is rich in fibrinogen and Factor VIII. It is not however free of the risk of non-A non-B hepatitis, and it contains the same degree of risk of infection with hepatitis B and HIV as other blood products, i.e. it depends on effective donor screening. It does appear to be useful in reversing the platelet defect in uraemia although the mechanism is unclear, but it is relatively deficient in Factor IX and is of no therapeutic value in haemophilia B.

54. B D

The bony destruction in multiple myeloma is believed to be a result of osteoclast activity due to the secretion of 'osteoclast activity factor' by the neoplastic cells. Bone healing is unusual even after a good response to therapy, and a compensatory increase in osteoblastic activity in response to therapy does not appear to occur: as a result bone scans are often unhelpful and the alkaline phosphatase remains normal despite occasionally markedly elevated serum calcium levels. IVPs are not contraindicated: the renal impairment associated with this procedure in myeloma in the past appears to result from deliberate dehydration prior to the IVP. Most patients die of infective complications. The value of the serum β_2 microglobulin level remains contentious but urinary levels are erratic and totally unhelpful. The serum level may be a prognostic indicator but a major factor in the elevation is renal impairment.

55. The following directly increase the anticoagulant effect of warfarin:

A aspirin
B barbiturates
C liver failure
D paracetamol
E heparin

Your answers: A.........B.........C.........D.........E.........

56. A bleeding diathesis due to

A idiopathic thrombocytopenic purpura (ITP) should be treated with platelet transfusion
B warfarin overdose should be treated with vitamin K intravenously
C massive blood transfusion should be treated with fresh frozen plasma (FFP) and platelet transfusion
D haemophilia, is accompanied by a positive Hess test
E von Willebrand's disease can be treated with desamino-D-arginine vasopressin (DDAVP)

Your answers: A.........B.........C.........D.........E.........

57. The following are features of iron-deficiency anaemia:

A reduced bone marrow stainable iron
B reduced serum iron and iron binding capacity (TIBC)
C a low MCV, MCH and MCHC
D target cells and pencil cells in the peripheral blood
E correction can almost always be achieved with simple oral iron preparations

Your answers: A.........B.........C.........D.........E.........

Answers overleaf

55. A C

Aspirin displaces protein bound warfarin and thereby increases the effect of orally administered warfarin on vitamin K dependent coagulation factors, as this drug is also protein bound. Barbiturates decrease the anticoagulant effect by enzyme induction and increasing warfarin destruction. Liver failure adds to the warfarin effect by reduction in factor production and impairment of vitamin K absorption. Paracetamol has no effect at normal dosage. Heparin does not directly affect warfarin's anticoagulant mechanism since it acts through enhanced antithrombin III activity, but it has an additive effect on anticoagulation.

56. C E

In ITP transfused platelets are rapidly coated with antibody and consumed in the same way as endogenously produced ones; they are of little value and of no value at all unless given in large quantities. Vitamin K reverses the warfarin effect too slowly to be of use if bleeding occurs. FFP should be used in this situation. Intravenous vitamin K renders subsequent warfarin dosage control very difficult. Stored blood contains few functional platelets, and has reduced V and VIII levels, so replacement with FFP and platelets is appropriate for bleeding secondary to massive blood transfusion. The Hess test is positive in situations where platelet numbers are low, platelets are poorly functional, or where there is undue vessel fragility; it is not positive in haemophilia. In mild haemophilia A and von Willebrand's disease, an intravenous bolus of DDAVP often causes a significant rise in circulating Factor VIII C and RAg and this is useful to cover bleeding episodes and minor operations.

57. C D E

Iron stores in the marrow have to be non-existent before any alteration in the Hb occurs; thereafter anaemia follows. Serum iron is reduced, but the TIBC increases, so that the TIBC is less than 10% saturated (viz. Fe/TIBC$\leqslant$1/10). The red cells are small, with reduced cell content and concentration, giving rise to the 'microcytic hypochromic' film which together with anisocytosis, target cells and pencil cells makes the classical iron deficiency picture. Oral iron is nearly always adequate; if the anaemia fails to respond, one should consider continued blood loss, severe malabsorption, poor compliance or a wrong initial diagnosis. Ferrous sulphate is the cheapest and most effective preparation.

58. The following are features of myelodysplastic syndrome:

A increased numbers of blasts in the bone marrow
B atypical monocytes in the peripheral blood
C transfusion-dependent anaemia
D transformation into treatment-resistant acute myeloid leukaemia (AML)
E treatment with busulphan may be effective

Your answers: A.........B.........C.........D.........E.........

59. Massive splenomegaly

A may cause pancytopenia
B may give rise to oesophageal varices
C may follow malaria
D may occur in kwashiorkor
E may result in relative polycythaemia due to a reduction in plasma volume

Your answers: A.........B.........C.........D.........E.........

60. In Hodgkin's disease

A impaired T-lymphocyte function is a recognised feature
B minimal change nephropathy may occur
C a history of spontaneous nodal shrinkage is unusual
D localised disease should be treated with local radiotherapy
E staging laparotomy is indicated prior to therapy

Your answers: A.........B.........C.........D.........E.........

Answers overleaf

58. A B C D

This heterogeneous group of conditions is usually characterised by transfusion-dependent, or 'refractory' anaemia. The presence of 5-20% blasts in the marrow is seen in refractory anaemia with excess of blasts. A proportion of patients transform into resistant AML, with a marrow blast count > 30%. A more indolent condition associated with atypical monocytes in the peripheral blood and marrow has been labelled 'chronic myelomonocytic leukaemia'. Treatment of these conditions with cytotoxic drugs prior to the development of frank leukaemia is of doubtful value. Busulphan is of value in the myeloproliferative disorders, not in this group of conditions.

59. A B C

Reduction in any or all of the blood cell lines may be secondary to splenomegaly, as may oesophageal varices on a purely haemodynamic basis. Malaria is the commonest cause of splenomegaly world-wide. Kwashiorkor results in abdominal distension due to hypoproteinaemic ascites; splenomegaly does not usually occur. An increased plasma volume is the normal finding in patients with significant splenomegaly.

60. A B

Tests of T-cell function are commonly abnormal in untreated Hodgkin's disease. Minimal change nephropathy is an uncommon but recognised complication and responds to treatment of the Hodgkin's disease. Variations within individual patients in the size of their lymphadenopathy are commonly reported. Extended radiotherapy (i.e. mantle or inverted Y but not local) is commonly administered. The value of a staging laparotomy is restricted to differentiating Stage IIA (disease above or below the diaphragm without constitutional upset) from Stage IIIA (disease above and below the diaphragm without constitutional upset). The former disease may be cured by radiation alone, whereas chemotherapy ± radiation is indicated for the latter.

61. Prostacyclin (PGI_2)

A is produced by platelets

B is the most powerful naturally occurring platelet inhibitor yet described

C acts in opposition to PGE_1

D inhibits platelet activity by the same mechanism as aspirin

E may be useful therapeutically by oral, intravenous or intra-arterial routes

Your answers: A.........B.........C.........D.........E.........

62. Heparin treatment for pulmonary embolus

A should be commenced as a constant intravenous infusion of 40,000 u/24 hours

B prolongs the prothrombin time (PT)

C may cause a fall in platelet count

D may give rise to osteomalacia

E if 'overdosed', may be reversed by quinine suphate

Your answers: A.........B.........C.........D.........E.........

63. In the normal neonate

A the white blood count may be $25 \times 10^9/l$

B haemoglobin F is the predominant haemoglobin

C the platelet count is in the normal adult range

D nucleated red cells are rarely seen in the peripheral blood

E the mean cell volume is greater than 100 fl

Your answers: A.........B.........C.........D.........E.........

Answers overleaf

61. B

PGI_2 is produced by many cells (endothelial cells in particular, also fibroblasts and macrophages) but not platelets which produce the vasoconstrictor and platelet activating thromboxane A_2 (TXA_2) by a parallel synthetic pathway. It is an extremely potent platelet inhibitor and vasodilator, exerting its effects by raising intraplatelet cyclic adenosine monophosphate (CAMP), unlike aspirin which acetylates and inactivates the enzyme cyclo-oxygenase and therefore prevents platelet production of TXA_2. PGE_1 has the same action but is less potent, it shares the same platelet receptor as PGI_2. Prostacyclin can be given by intravenous and intra-arterial routes but not orally.

62. B C

The starting dose should be weight-related, (25 u/kg/hour); a 'standard' starting dose will frequently result in over- or underdosage. Heparin's chief action is to promote anti-thrombin III's inactivation of thrombin and therefore to prolong the PT, and kaolin cephalin clotting time (KCCT). KCTT is normally used to control therapy. Prolonged heparin treatment can give rise to thrombocytopenia (within weeks) and osteoporosis (within months, e.g. during pregnancy). Protamine sulphate (1 mg neutralises 100 u of heparin) in a dose of 1 mg/100 u heparin may be used to reverse the effect of heparin in vitro and in vivo.

63. A B C E

The full blood count in the normal neonate is quite different from the normal adult one. Most neonates have a WBC count between 9- 30×10^9/l and 'elevated' levels persist for several weeks. At birth neutrophils predominate in the differential WBC. Nucleated red cells are commonly present. The MCV is high, and remains above adult levels for at least 2 months. Haemoglobin F remains the major haemoglobin until about 3 months.

64. ß-thalassaemia major

A may present with severe anaemia between the ages of 5 and 10 years
B commonly presents with neonatal jaundice
C can be diagnosed antenatally by Hb electrophoresis on fetal red cells
D is associated with splenic atrophy in older patients
E should be treated with regular oral desferrioxamine to reduce iron overload

Your answers: A.........B.........C.........D.........E.........

65. In allogeneic bone marrow transplant for acute leukaemia

A the donor must be of the same ABO blood group
B the survival figures are no better for patients grafted in remission compared with those in relapse
C graft versus host disease (GVHD) is rare if the donor and recipient are matched at the HLA A, B and DR loci, and unreactive in mixed lymphocyte culture
D total body irradiation (TBI) is effective in reducing the severity of GVHD
E GVHD reduces the risk of subsequent relapse

Your answers: A.........B.........C.........D.........E.........

66. When giving a blood transfusion

A administration of Rhesus positive blood to a Rhesus positive recipient can be followed by haemolytic problems due to Rhesus-group antibodies
B a fever in the recipient developing during transfusion is an indication to stop transfusing
C using stored blood, the oxygen delivering capacity of the blood is not restored until around 2 days later
D prior transfusion with dextran may give rise to a transfusion reaction
E with stored blood, one can assume that no viable white blood cells remain 24 hours after the blood donation.

Your answers: A.........B.........C.........D.........E.........

Answers overleaf

64. None are correct

ß thalassaemia major by definition presents within the first year of life after the switch to Hb A, as production of the latter is severely impaired. Due to normal production of embryonic and fetal haemoglobins, the diagnosis cannot be made antenatally on fetal red cell electrophoresis, but requires family DNA studies. For the same reason the neonate is not affected and jaundice does not result. Splenomegaly occurs progressively and splenectomy is usually undertaken to reduce transfusion requirements. Oral desferrioxamine is not absorbed satisfactorily, and to achieve a reduction in raised body iron consequent upon increased iron absorption and transfusion requires parenteral chelation.

65. E

ABO incompatibility is not a contraindication to transplant, and necessitates only red cell depletion from the graft to prevent haemolytic reactions. The results of allogeneic transplant carried out in first complete remission are much better than those in relapse. GVHD often occurs in patients 'fully matched' with their donors (up to 70% prior to T- cell depletion) presumably due to unrecognised minor histocompatibility groups, and is not reduced following TBI, indeed it may be worse. There is a clear reduction in relapse of disease in patients who have significant GVHD: the so-called 'graft-versus-leukaemia' effect.

66. A

The term 'Rhesus positive' refers to patients whose red cells bear the antigen 'D', and does not take account of the other antigens in the Rhesus group. Thus 'Rhesus positive' blood which is commonly CDe/cde may induce antibody formation against C, c or e if the recipient does not possess these antigens. Fever may develop during transfusion due to non-specific pyrogens or to WBC or platelet antibodies in patients who have received previous transfusions; it is safe to continue *as long as* no additional signs and symptoms develop. 2,3-diphosphoglycerate is reduced in stored red cells, but is restored 4-12 hours after transfusion thus restoring oxygen delivering capacity. Dextran infusion can cause RBC agglutination in vitro and so complicate the cross-match reaction. It does not cause clinical problems. Lymphocytes remain viable in stored blood for several days and can cause 'graft versus host' disease in severely immuno-compromised recipients

67. The following are in keeping with a diagnosis of severe iron deficiency anaemia:

A early introduction of mixed feeding in an infant
B haemosiderinuria
C low plasma haptoglobin
D splenomegaly
E painful red tongue

Your answers: A.........B.........C.........D.........E.........

68. In chronic granulocytic leukaemia (CGL)

A a 9,22 chromosome translocation is necessary to establish the diagnosis
B transformation into myelofibrosis may occur
C development of further chromosome abnormalities heralds a change in the character of the disease
D busulphan therapy delays the onset of blast transformation
E bone marrow transplantation in chronic phase may be curative

Your answers: A.........B.........C.........D.........E.........

69. Fanconi's anaemia (FA)

A is associated with hyperpigmentation in most patients
B is inherited as an autosomal dominant disorder
C is characteristically associated with a hypochromic microcytic red cell appearance
D commonly presents as aplastic anaemia soon after birth
E has a uniformly poor prognosis without bone marrow transplantation (BMT)

Your answers: A.........B.........C.........D.........E.........

Answers overleaf

67. E

Delayed mixed feeding is a frequent cause of infantile iron deficiency due to low iron content in human and cows' milk. A mucositis is a common feature of IDA with a painful red smooth tongue, and gastritis may also occur. Haemosiderinuria is a feature of chronic intravascular haemolysis. A low plasma haptoglobin is a feature of intravascular haemolysis. Splenomegaly should not be regarded as simply a result of iron deficiency, in practice it is rarely if ever solely due to this.

68. B C E

Whilst a 9,22 chromosome translocation resulting in the classical 'Philadelphia' chromosome is the usual finding, more complex abnormalities involving a third chromosome are not uncommon and Philadelphia negative CGL with evidence of the same specific molecular DNA rearrangement is now recognised. Acceleration of the disease course with transformation into acute leukaemia or myelofibrosis is often preceded by new chromosomal abnormalities such as loss of the Y chromosome, altered chromosome 17 and others. Although busulphan controls the leukocytosis, conventional chemotherapy like this does not appear to delay the onset of the accelerated phase. However, bone marrow transplantation may be curative if carried out before disease acceleration occurs.

69. A E

Hyperpigmentation is a characteristic feature of FA, occurring in 77% of cases. Inheritance is autosomal recessive and the red cells are usually macrocytic. Although skeletal and renal abnormalities are frequently detected soon after birth, anaemia usually develops between 5 and 10 years of age. The prognosis is extremely poor. Anabolic steroids may produce an improvement in the blood count, but this is generally incomplete and transient and without BMT most patients die within 4 years of diagnosis.

INFECTIOUS DISEASES

Indicate your answers by putting T (True), F (False) or D (Don't know) in the spaces provided.

70. Eosinophilia usually occurs in

A schistosomiasis
B taenia saginatum
C malaria
D filariasis
E amoebiasis (*Entamoeba histolytica*)

Your answers: A.........B.........C.........D.........E.........

71. Hepatitis A infection

A is usually subclinical or anicteric
B incidence increases in the winter and autumn
C does not lead to chronic active hepatitis
D is a sexually transmissible disease
E generally confers lasting immunity

Your answers: A.........B.........C.........D.........E.........

72. In typhoid fever

A rose spots appear in the third week
B headache is common
C cholecystectomy prolongs carriage
D stool culture is most likely to be positive in the first week of the illness
E antibiotic treatment prolongs carriage

Your answers: A.........B.........C.........D.........E.........

Answers overleaf

70. A B D

Metazoan (multicellular) parasites, which include nematodes such as *Wuchereria bancrofti* (filariasis), trematodes such as the *Schistosoma*, and cestodes such as *Taenia saginata*, cause eosinophilia during tissue invasion or migration. Protozoan (unicellular) parasites, such as *Plasmodium* species (malaria) and *Entamoeba histolytica* (amoebiasis), do not cause eosinophilia.

71. A B C D E

Hepatitis A infection is frequently subclinical or articteric, particularly in children in whom the illness is usually milder and has a shorter duration. Chronic hepatitis is a well recognised consequence of hepatitis B and non-A non-B hepatitis, but not hepatitis A. Although spread is usually by the faecal-oral route, hepatitis A may be spread by sexual intercourse or parenterally. After acute infection hepatitis A antibodies of IgG class remain detectable indefinitely, and patients with serum antibodies are immune to infection.

72. B

The diagnosis of typhoid relies in the first week on the clinical features including headache, malaise, anorexia and fever, and on blood cultures. The characteristic rash (rose spots) is most often observed in the second week of the disease. Stool culture is unlikely to be positive until the second or third week. Chronic carriage may be associated with gallbladder disease but antibiotic treatment, as well as being used to treat the acute illness, is also sometimes used to treat chronic carriers.

73. In viral hepatitis

A delta virus infection occurs only in the presence of hepatitis B virus
B non-A non-B is the commonest transfusion associated hepatitis in developed countries
C anti-Hbs usually appears during the acute phase of the illness
D the incubation period for non-A non-B hepatitis is less than 6 weeks
E anti-HBc is detectable before anti-HBs

Your answers: A.........B.........C.........D.........E.........

74. Examination of the sputum is usually diagnostic in

A mycoplasma pneumonia
B paragonomiasis
C aspergilloma
D pneumococcal pneumonia
E pneumocystic pneumonia

Your answers: A.........B.........C.........D.........E.........

75. Herpes viruses

A may be associated with nasopharyngeal carcinoma
B are RNA viruses
C may be distinguished from one another by electron microscopy
D can cross the placenta
E are latent viruses

Your answers: A.........B.........C.........D.........E.........

Answers overleaf

73. A B E

Delta virus is an incomplete virus which requires the presence of hepatitis B virus for replication. Non-A non-B hepatitis may have an incubation period up to 150 days. It is not possible to screen blood donors for non-A non-B hepatitis unlike hepatitis B. In hepatitis B infection, titres of anti-HBc rise during the acute phase of the illness, but decline to a low titre following recovery. Anti-HBs titres do not rise until some weeks or months after anti-HBc.

74. B D

Microscopic examination of sputum will usually distinguish pneumococcal and staphylococcal pneumonia from that due to Gram-negative organisms which require different antibiotic treatment. *Mycoplasma* is rarely cultured from sputum and diagnosis relies on serological tests. The finding of *Aspergillus* in the sputum also occurs in bronchopulmonary aspergillosis. The eggs of *Paragonimus* in the lung are expectorated and hence diagnosis is made by examining the sputum. Transbronchial lung biopsy or bronchoalveolar lavage is generally required to diagnose pneumonia due to *Pneumocystis carinii.*

75. A D E

The herpes viruses are DNA viruses, and include varicella-zoster, herpes simplex, cytomegalovirus and Epstein-Barr virus. They cannot be distinguished by electron microscopy but they differ in clinical, serological and cytopathic effects. As well as crossing the placenta to cause some congenital defects, they also lie dormant after the initial infection and can cause further problems particularly if the host becomes immunocompromised. Recent studies have suggested an association between Epstein-Barr virus and Burkitt's lymphoma and nasopharyngeal carcinoma.

76. Legionnaires' disease

A is caused by a Gram-positive bacillus
B is often spread from person to person
C is commoner in winter and spring
D produces signs on chest examination that are more marked than the chest X-ray appearances
E is associated with hyponatraemia

Your answers: A.........B.........C.........D.........E.........

77. In tuberculosis

A acid-fast bacilli (AFB) are found on microscopy of CSF deposits in most cases of TB meningitis
B tuberculin testing generally becomes positive about 6 weeks after the onset of the primary infection
C viable mycobacteria disappear from the sputum after a few days of effective chemotherapy
D neonatal BCG vaccination is ineffective
E systemic features are often lacking in tuberculous lymphadenitis

Your answers: A.........B.........C.........D.........E.........

78. The following are true about rashes:

A the rash associated with infectious mononucleosis may appear without antibiotics being prescribed
B the rash of scabies is rarely found above the neck in adults
C almost all patients with meningococcal septicaemia develop a purpuric rash
D erythema marginatum is associated with streptococcal sensitisation
E the rash of measles usually appears first on the trunk

Your answers: A.........B.........C.........D.........E.........

Answers overleaf

76. E

Legionella pneumophila is a poorly staining Gram-negative rod that is difficult to grow in vitro. Spread by person to person contact is not recognised. The excess of Legionnaires' disease in the summer is largely due to travel-associated cases. As with other atypical pneumonias the ill patient may have few chest signs. Hyponatraemia is frequently found and may be due to inappropriate secretion of antidiuretic hormone.

77. B C E

In tuberculous meningitis AFB can be identified in about 25% of CSF deposits but culture will be positive in the majority. After primary infection tuberculis conversion generally occurs within six weeks, but may take up to 3 months in some. In pulmonary tuberculosis effective multiple drug chemotherapy rapidly sterilises the sputum. BCG vaccination at, or shortly after birth, is safe and provides some protection for at least 10 years. Tuberculous lymphadenitis (scrofula) often occurs in the absence of other symptoms.

78. A B D

Although the rash in infectious mononucleosis is most commonly secondary to antibiotic treatment, the disease itself may produce a rash. Scabies affects many parts of the body but usually spares the face and scalp. Only about 50% of cases of meningococcal septicaemia have the characteristic rash. Erythema marginatum is a major criterion in the diagnosis of rheumatic fever. The measles rash begins on the neck and spreads to the face and trunk.

79. Live vaccines are used in immunisation against the following diseases:

A tuberculosis
B hepatitis B
C diphtheria
D rubella
E yellow fever

Your answers: A.........B.........C.........D.........E.........

80. In Lassa fever

A the incubation period is between 28 and 40 days
B the virus can be isolated from the urine
C the vector is a flea
D the disease is endemic in East Africa
E the disease is usually fatal

Your answers: A.........B.........C.........D.........E.........

81. Immunoglobulins may be useful in post-exposure prophylaxis in the following conditions:

A chickenpox
B hepatitis B
C rabies
D tetanus
E whooping cough

Your answers: A.........B.........C.........D.........E.........

Answers overleaf

79. A D E

BCG vaccination employs a live attenuated strain of *Mycobacterium bovis*, Bacillus Calmette-Guérin. Current hepatitis B vaccine uses surface antigen rather than whole virus and diphtheria toxoid is used for immunisation. Live attenuated viruses are used for rubella and yellow fever. It is recommended that an interval of three weeks is left between any two live vaccines. If time does not permit, the two live vaccines should be given at the same time (at different sites), rather than at a shorter interval.

80. B

The virus which causes Lassa fever is an arenavirus which can be isolated from the urine, blood or throat washings of an infected person. The disease is endemic in West Aftica, where wild rodents act as a reservoir, transmitting the disease probably via infected urine, though person to person spread does occur. Mortality in epidemics approaches 50% but subclinical infection is common in endemic areas. The incubation period is no greater than 21 days.

81. A B C D

Zoster immune globulin (ZIG) is available to protect immunocompromised individuals, especially children, against chickenpox. Specific immunoglobulins against hepatitis B, rabies and tetanus are given to people who may have been exposed to infection, and a course of vaccination is often commenced at the same time. There is no specific therapy available for post-exposure prophylaxis of whooping cough, although antibiotic therapy may possibly be of value if given at an early stage of the illness.

82. In falciparum malaria

A steroids may be helpful when treating cerebral malaria
B quinine is the treatment of choice in chloroquine-resistant areas
C primaquine must be given after chloroquine treatment
D in chloroquine sensitive areas proguanil is an effective alternative chemoprophylactic agent
E the male mosquito transmits the disease

Your answers: A.........B.........C.........D.........E.........

83. Infectious mononucleosis may cause

A mild or inapparent infection in childhood
B a palpably enlarged spleen in about 50% of cases
C thrombocytosis
D a rash in most patients
E a facial palsy

Your answers: A.........B.........C.........D.........E.........

84. The following may be associated with hepatic granulomata:

A sarcoidosis
B malaria
C cytomegalovirus
D echinococcus (hydatid disease)
E syphilis

Your answers: A.........B.........C.........D.........E.........

Answers overleaf

82. B D

Steroid therapy has traditionally been used in the treatment of cerebral malaria, but it is of no value and may even be harmful. Primaquine therapy is used to prevent relapse in malaria due to the liver forms of *P. vivax* and *P. ovale; P. falciparum* does not have liver forms. Proguanil is given in a daily dosage and is used only as a prophylactic agent. Malaria is transmitted by the female anopheline mosquito.

83. A B E

Lymphadenopathy is usually present at some stage of the illness and the spleen is palpable in about half the cases. Rare complications include thrombocytopenia, haemolytic anaemia, myocarditis, pericarditis, lymphocytic meningitis, encephalitis and polyneuritis. The rash sometimes seen in infectious mononucleosis is nearly always due to antibiotics and only rarely does the disease itself produce a rash. Subclinical infection in childhood is common.

84. A C E

Infection with cytomegalovirus may occur in healthy adults, as well as the immunosuppressed, and commonly causes granulomatous hepatitis as well as mononucleosis. Sarcoidosis may affect many organs and the clinical manifestations depend on the site, the degree of granulomatous activity, and secondary fibrosis. Granulomas due to syphilis (gumma) occur late in the disease and can develop in any organ. Although malaria and hydatid disease may affect the liver, they are not associated with the formation of granulomata.

85. The following complications are associated with these drugs:

A haemolysis and penicillin
B retinopathy and isoniazid
C renal failure and tetracyclines
D peripheral neuropathy and metronidazole
E hepatitis and chloroquine

Your answers: A.........B.........C.........D.........E.........

86. The clinical features in these diseases are mediated by a toxin

A diphtheria
B giardiasis
C pseudomembranous colitis
D poliomyelitis
E toxocariasis

Your answers: A.........B.........C.........D.........E.........

87. The following diseases have an insect vector:

A Lassa fever
B onchocerciasis
C schistosomiasis
D trypanosomiasis
E cysticercosis

Your answers: A.........B.........C.........D.........E.........

Answers overleaf

85. A C D

Haemolysis may be associated with a variety of antibiotics including penicillins, sulphonamides, cephalosporins, isoniazid and rifampicin. Isoniazid may cause a peripheral neuropathy or hepatitis, whereas chloroquine can cause a retinopathy. In general tetracyclines may exacerbate renal failure and should not be given to patients with renal disease. Long-term usage of metronidazole can lead to a peripheral neuropathy.

86. A C

The systemic features of clinical diphtheria are entirely accounted for by the diphtheria toxin, and they do not occur with infection by non- toxigenic strains. The widespread use of diphtheria toxoid has lead to the control of this disease. Although toxins are implicated in the pathogenesis of many infectious diarrhoeas including *Clostridium difficile* in pseudomembranous colitis, there is no evidence of toxin production by *Giardia lamblia*. The polio virus directly affects the anterior horn cells and the clinical features of toxocara result from larval migration.

87. B D

Lassa fever is transmitted by direct or indirect contact with the urine of infected rodents in dust or on food, but has no known insect vector. Schistosomiasis requires the snail as an intermediate host, but does not have an insect vector. Cysticercosis is due to infection with eggs of *Taenia solium* acquired by contact with contaminated human faeces. Onchocerciasis is transmitted by blackflies and trypanosomiasis by the tsetse fly in Africa and the reduvid bug in South America.

88. The following worm infestations enter the human via the skin:

A *Ascaris lumbricoides*
B *Strongyloides stercoralis*
C *Trichuris trichiura*
D *Ancylostoma duodenale*
E *Dracunculus*

Your answers: A.........B.........C.........D.........E.........

89. The following are recognised complications of measles:

A otitis media
B facial palsy
C pancreatitis
D subacute sclerosing panencephalitis (SSPE)
E staphylococcal pneumonia

Your answers: A.........B.........C.........D.........E.........

90. The following diseases are notifiable in England and Wales:

A whooping cough
B brucellosis
C malaria
D rubella
E acute meningitis

Your answers: A.........B.........C.........D.........E.........

Answers overleaf

88. B D

The larvae of *Ancylostoma* and *Strongyloides* penetrate the skin, usually via the foot, to continue their life-cycles in man. Ascariasis and trichuriasis are the most prevalent helminthic infections in man: both require ingestion of their eggs, which are excreted in human faeces, for transmission. Dracunculiasis (guinea worm infection) develops after drinking water containing copepods (crustaceans) infected with *Dracunculus.*

89. A D E

Secondary bacterial infections play a large part in the respiratory tract complications of measles which include otitis media, laryngitis, bronchitis and pneumonia. Staphylococci may be responsible for pneumonia after measles, but streptococci and *Haemophilus influenzae* are also commonly seen. Central nervous system complications of measles include convulsions, encephalitis and very rarely SSPE. Cranial nerve palsies are not a feature, and pancreatitis is a complication of mumps.

90. A C E

The system of statutory notification was created to facilitate the local control of infectious diseases, and also provide information for national surveillance. Medical practitioners should notify the names and addresses of people recognised as, or suspected of, having any of the specified illnesses to the local Medical Officer for Environmental Health (MOEH). Not all infectious diseases are notifiable e.g. brucellosis and rubella. Despite significant under-notification the system provides valuable information on trends in disease incidence.

91. In leprosy

A neural lesions generally appear earlier than dermal lesions in the lepromatous type

B erythema nodosum leprosum commonly occurs in tuberculoid leprosy

C infection via the respiratory tract is the most likely route of infection with *Mycobacterium leprae*

D the lepromin test is usually positive in lepromatous leprosy

E dapsone alone is no longer considered the treatment of choice for any form of leprosy

Your answers: A.........B.........C.........D.........E.........

92. In leptospirosis

A the disease is more common in winter than summer

B nephritis is a common accompaniment

C cattle form an important source of the illness in man

D blood cultures do not become positive until the second week

E penicillin or tetracycline are the treatments of choice early in the disease

Your answers: A.........B.........C.........D.........E.........

93. In rickettsial diseases

A the Weil-Felix reaction is negative in 'Q' fever

B the louse is the vector in Rocky Mountain Spotted Fever

C 'Q' fever is a recognised cause of protracted hepatitis

D the mammalian host is the rat in epidemic typhus

E recrudescent typhus (Brill-Zinsser disease) occurs with *Rickettsia prowazeki*

Your answers: A.........B.........C.........D.........E.........

Answers overleaf

91. C E

Neural lesions generally appear earlier in the tuberculoid type of leprosy; dermal lesions are more numerous in the lepromatous type. Erythema nodosum leprosum is a most troublesome complication that occurs only in cases at the lepromatous end of the spectrum. The lepromin test is negative in the lepromatous type, but usually positive in the tuberculoid type. Although skin to skin spread is thought to occur in leprosy, the presence of large numbers of mycobacteria in nasal secretions is believed to be the main source of infection. Dapsone is usually combined with rifampicin in the initial stages of treatment (plus clofazimine in the lepromatous type).

92. B C E

The increased incidence of leptospirosis in the summer and early autumn probably results from indirect contact with infected urine via contaminated recreational waters. Dogs, cattle, rodents, cats, and other wild mammals are the important sources of illness in man. Interstitial nephritis is the basic lesion in human leptospiral illness. The organism is usually cultured from the blood in the first week of the illness and in the urine thereafter. Antibiotic treatment is probably ineffective if given after the first week of illness.

93. A C E

The Weil-Felix reaction is positive in a variety of rickettsial diseases, including epidemic (louse-borne) and endemic (murine) typhus, and Rocky Mountain Spotted Fever, but the louse is the vector in epidemic typhus where the human is the mammalian host. *Rickettsia prowazeki* causes epidemic typhus, and the recrudescent form, Brill-Zinsser disease.

94. When immunising

A polio vaccination need not be repeated after childhood
B measles vaccination is usually given at 3 months
C whooping cough vaccination is contraindicated during a febrile illness
D tetanus vaccination should be repeated every 3 years in adults
E rubella vaccine is contraindicated in individuals with a past history of the illness.

Your answers: A.........B.........C.........D.........E.........

95. In poliomyelitis

A epidemics are associated with a large number of asymptomatic excretors
B physical exertion may predispose to paralysis
C the paralysis is accompanied by sensory changes
D the disease may present as an aseptic meningitis
E bulbar paralysis may contribute to the respiratory problems

Your answers: A.........B.........C.........D.........E.........

96. The following statements about acute respiratory tract infections are correct:

A influenza A virus is responsible for world pandemics
B measles virus is a common cause of acute obstructive laryngitis (croup)
C acute epiglottitis is commonly due to *Haemophilus influenzae*
D in diphtheria the treatment of choice is penicillin
E parainfluenza virus is responsible for most cases of bronchiolitis in infants

Your answers: A.........B.........C.........D.........E.........

Answers overleaf

94. C

It is recommended that a reinforcing dose of polio vaccine be given to 15-19 year olds on leaving school or before employment. Further reinforcing doses are not necessary for adults unless they are at special risk of contracting the disease e.g. by travelling to countries where polio is endemic. Maternal antibodies generally protect against measles during infancy and the vaccine is usually given in the second year of life. Whooping cough vaccination is contraindicated during an acute febrile illness and should be delayed until full recovery. Tetanus vaccines should not be given to anyone who has received a booster in the last five years. History is an unreliable indicator of previous rubella infection, and vaccination in the presence of immunity is safe.

95. A B D E

Polio infection spreads by the faecal-oral route and during epidemics there may be many asymptomatic excretors. Factors which predispose to paralysis include pregnancy, tonsillectomy, prophylactic injections and physical exertion. The virus affects the anterior horn cells and consequently is not accompanied by sensory changes. Polio may present as an acute illness with pyrexia, headache, vomiting and signs of meningeal irritation. In addition to respiratory muscle paralysis, bulbar paralysis may cause aspiration, and the respiratory centre may be affected directly.

96. A B C

World pandemics may occur if there is a major antigenic shift in the influenza A virus which produces a new viral strain to which the general population possesses no immunity. Influenza B and C viruses have not been responsible for pandemics. Croup may be caused by a variety of viruses, but parainfluenza virus and measles virus are the most common. *Haemophilus influenzae* is isolated from most patients with acute epiglottitis, but other bacteria are occasionally implicated. The role of viruses in epiglottitis is not established. The mainstay of treatment in diphtheria is antitoxin, though antibiotics may help reduce bacterial numbers. Respiratory syncitial virus is the commonest cause of bronchiolitis in infants.

97. In meningitis

A steroids are useful in the prevention of neurological sequelae of acute bacterial meningitis

B due to *Mycobacterium tuberculosis* the CSF sugar is normal

C in neonates, group B haemolytic streptococcus is a common cause

D ampicillin is a suitable prophylactic agent for contacts of patients with meningococcal meningitis

E *Staphylococcus aureus* is the commonest cause in patients with ventriculo-atrial shunts

Your answers: A.........B.........C.........D.........E.........

98. The following signs are found in secondary syphilis:

A iritis

B lymphadenopathy

C condylomata acuminata

D alopecia

E urethral discharge

Your answers: A.........B.........C.........D.........E.........

99. Delayed hypersensitivity may be impaired in

A sarcoidosis

B tuberculosis

C Hodgkin's disease

D Bruton's syndrome (X-linked hypogammaglobulinaemia)

E di George's syndrome (thymus aplasia)

Your answers: A.........B.........C.........D.........E.........

Answers overleaf

97. C

Steroids have not been shown to be beneficial in the treatment of acute bacterial meningitis. CSF sugar is usually reduced in tuberculous meningitis and normal in viral meningitis. In neonatal meningitis the infection probably originates from the genital tract of the mother and other commonly encountered organisms include *E. coli* and *Listeria monocytogenes*. Although penicillins are used in the treatment of acute meningococcal meningitis, they are ineffective as prophylactic agents. *Staphylococcus epidermidis* and Gram-negative bacilli are the usual shunt-associated infections.

98. A B D

Syphilis is known as the 'great imitator'. Secondary, or disseminated, syphilis describes the most clinically florid stage of the infection and occurs 2-8 weeks after the appearance of the primary chancre. It has a myriad of symptoms and signs, of which the most commonly recognised are the skin lesions including a rash, condylomata lata (flat warts), and alopecia. Many other organs may be affected, including the eyes, but urethral discharge is not a feature. Painless lymphadenopathy is also common and this classically includes the epitrochlear nodes.

99. A B C E

T cell function is reflected in the delayed hypersensitivity reaction which can be tested using common antigens such as purified protein derivative (PPD). A negative tuberculin skin test is characteristic of sarcoidosis, and may be impaired in severe tuberculosis. T lymphocyte responses may be impaired in Hodgkin's disease and in di George's syndrome (a congenital maldevelopment affecting the parathyroids and thymus). T cell function is not affected in Bruton's syndrome, where the abnormality lies in the production of immunoglobulins.

100. The following are true of the Acquired Immunodeficiency Syndrome (AIDS):

A it is a notifiable disease
B *Pneumocystis carinii* pneumonia has a characteristic X-ray appearance
C diarrhoea due to cryptosporidium responds to metronidazole
D it may lead to presenile dementia
E it cannot be diagnosed without a positive serological test

Your answers: A.........B.........C.........D.........E.........

101. In infective endocarditis

A finger clubbing is a frequent feature
B a previously normal valve may be affected
C in drug addicts the tricuspid valve is often involved
D the RA Latex test is often positive
E with prosthetic valves *Candida* is a frequent pathogen

Your answers: A.........B.........C.........D.........E.........

102. In schistosomiasis

A the adult worms multiply in man
B complete immunity follows initial infection
C the disease can be diagnosed by rectal biopsy
D oesophageal varices are a recognised complication
E oxamniquine is used to treat *Schistosoma japonicum*

Your answers: A.........B.........C.........D.........E.........

Answers overleaf

100. D

AIDS remains a clinical diagnosis and hence does not rely on serological tests for the Human Immunodeficiency Virus (HIV). Chest X-ray changes are similar for a variety of opportunistic infections and are not therefore diagnostic. There is at present no effective drug available to treat cryptosporidium. Encephalopathy and early dementia may result directly from HIV infection or from opportunists like cytomegalovirus. In the United Kingdom neither infection with HIV, nor the diagnosis of AIDS, are statutorily notifiable. However voluntary reporting of cases is encouraged to the Communicable Disease Surveillance Centre, where a confidential register is maintained.

101. B C D E

Finger clubbing is a late feature and rarely seen now in association with endocarditis. Although abnormal valves may be more susceptible to infection, any normal valve can be affected. Left sided lesions are most common but intravenous drug abusers are at risk of tricuspid lesions as this valve is the first to 'meet' injected contaminated material. Rheumatoid factor develops in about half of patients with infective endocarditis of more than six weeks duration; most patients become negative again after therapy. Candidal endocarditis affects prosthetic valves, and may occur in drug addicts and after prolonged antibiotic therapy.

102. C D

Each adult worm may produce many eggs, but the total worm load carried by an individual is increased only by repeated infection. *Schistosoma mansonii, S. japonicum* and *S. haematobium* ova may all be observed on rectal biopsy, and eggs may also be seen in stool samples (or urine in the case of *S. haematobium*). Oxamniquine is used to treat *S. mansoni*, but praziquantel is effective against all the main human schistosome species, including *S. japonicum*.

REVISION INDEX

Each item in this index refers to a specific question or answer. The numbers given refer to question numbers not page numbers.